Cooking with Wheat

What are Wheat Berries?

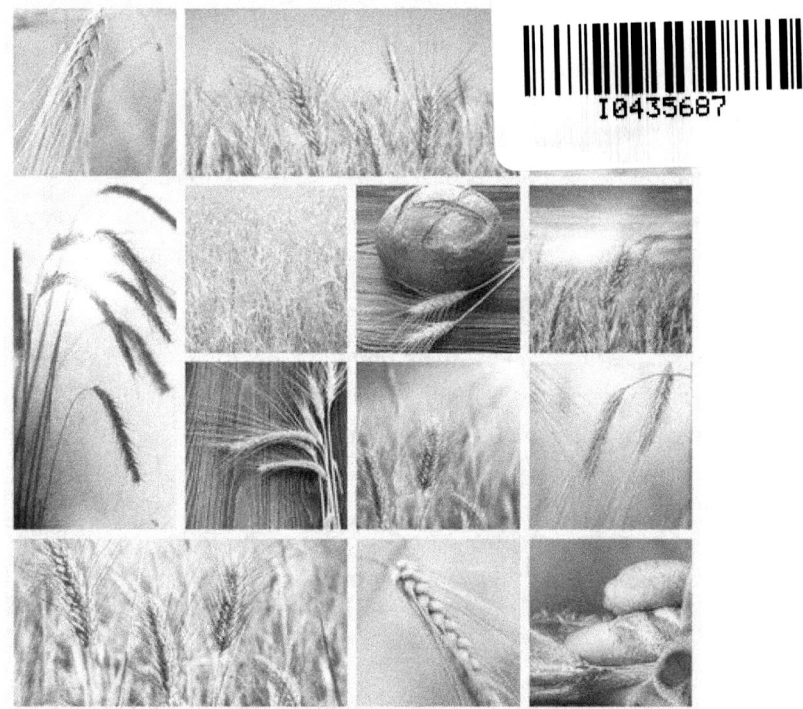

Healthy Cooking Series

Dueep J. Singh

Mendon Cottage Books

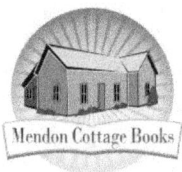

JD-Biz Publishing

Disclaimer

The information is this book is provided for informational purposes only. It is not intended to be used and medical advice or a substitute for proper medical treatment by a qualified health care provider. The information is believed to be accurate as presented based on research by the author.

The contents have not been evaluated by the U.S. Food and Drug Administration or any other Government or Health Organization and the contents in this book are not to be used to treat cure or prevent disease.

The author or publisher is not responsible for the use or safety of any diet, procedure or treatment mentioned in this book. The author or publisher is not responsible for errors or omissions that may exist.

Warning

The Book is for informational purposes only and before taking on any diet, treatment or medical procedure, it is recommended to consult with your primary health care provider.

Check out some of the other Healthy Gardening Series books at Amazon.com

Gardening Series on Amazon

Check out some of the other Health Learning Series books at Amazon.com

Health Learning Series on Amazon

Table of Contents

Introduction... 4

What Is a Wheat "Berry" 7

Nutritional Specifications of Wheat............................... 9

The difference between parboiled And Cracked Wheat 10

Our Daily Bread.. 12

Plain White Bread... 15

How Do You Get the Right Flour Consistency?...................................... 19

Shaping the Dough.. 22

Making Plaits 23

Dinner Rolls 23

Mini cottage loaves 24

Testing the bread.. 24

Making a Cheese Loaf 25

Perfect Bread Tips... 26

More Traditional Wheat Dishes 26

Bulgur Pilaf.. 28

Tabbouleh- Tabouli Salad 30

Frumenty 32

Cous-cous.. 33

Appendix.. 34

Traditional Chicken Soup 34

Panjiri- Pinnis... 36

Conclusion 38

Author Bio- 39

Publisher 49

Introduction

When man decided more than 10,000 years ago that he had had enough of having a life as a hunter and wanted to settle down as a farmer, that was a signal change in the history of mankind.

Prehistoric history does not tell us where man first began cultivating cereals as a grain for his family and for the people of his settlement. But archaeological excavations have found vestiges of this cultivated plant in settlements more than 10,000 years old in the Mesopotamian region. I would not be surprised if this wild grass was first cultivated in the area, especially near the river Tigris, Syria, Iraq, Lebanon, Babylon, etc.

After that, the cultivation of this particular wild grass, in the form of wheat spread all over the world, including Europe, Asia, Africa, – especially Egypt, where this grain was brewed into beer and drunk in large quantities by Pharoah and peasant alike millenniums ago – Turkey and all the places where there were hungry mouths to feed, and there were fertile lands to provide that grain to feed them.

This book introduces you to one of these most prolific and healthy cereals – wheat.

Wheat in its original form was a wild grass. Down the ages, it began to get domesticated, and the grains grew larger. Instead of being harvested by the wind in its wild form, the grains stayed attached to spikelets, until the farmer came with his scythe to harvest a rich crop of golden wheat.

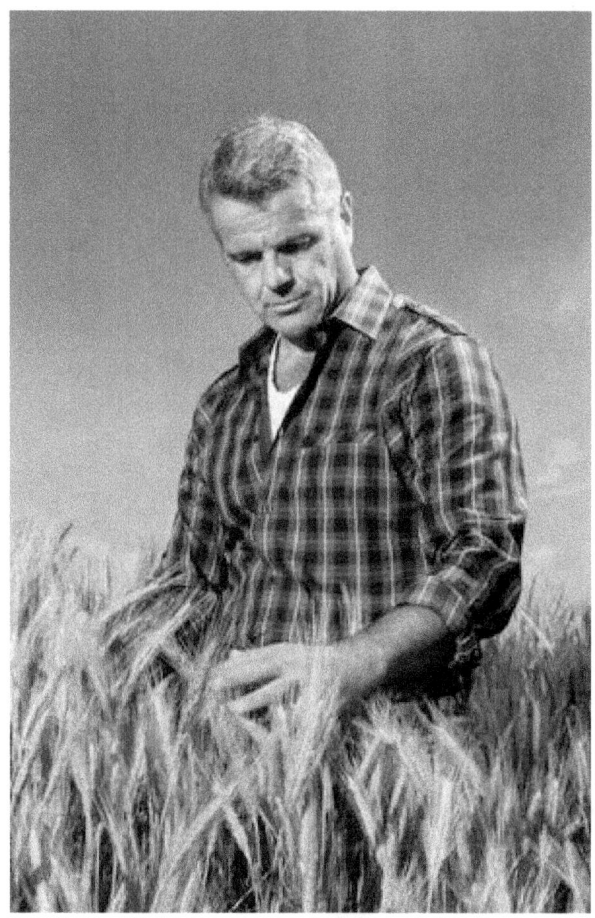

This was the grain, on which cities rose and economies flourished for millenniums. No wonder, the wheat grain was so precious a part of the social fabric, that it was worshiped, especially when the Greek goddess Demeter was always seen with a sheaf of wheat grain. She was also called Ceres or the Goddess of Agriculture. From her comes the term Cere-al for those precious grains of wheat.

The granaries of Egyptian pharaohs, Babylonian and Assyrian kings, Persian satraps, and emperors and chieftains of the east overflowed with wheat, which was produced in the rich and fertile lands of well irrigated countryside.

Even today, wheat is still being preserved in the ancient manner in airtight granaries before it is exported all over the world or sold in the local market.

When wheat was a wild grass, the rachis used to be fragile. It broke off very easily, and the seeds attached to the spikelets could be scattered on the ground. And so these seeds could cover more areas, through the dispersal mediums of natural methods like air, and water. But down the ages wheat is one of the cereals which has become more or less domesticated, like rice, barley and oats.

The wheat that we sow in our fields, today is a much more evolved and mutated variety, than the wheat grown more than 10,000 years ago. And thanks to this evolution, we can gather seeds more easily, but the natural dispersal trait of this once wild grass has disappeared during this course of evolution. That is why domesticated and mutated strains of wheat cannot flourish in the wild because they need to be harvested by hand.

What Is a Wheat "Berry"

A wheat berry – wheat berry – is the term being used for just an ordinary kernel of wheat, which has been taken out from the husk.

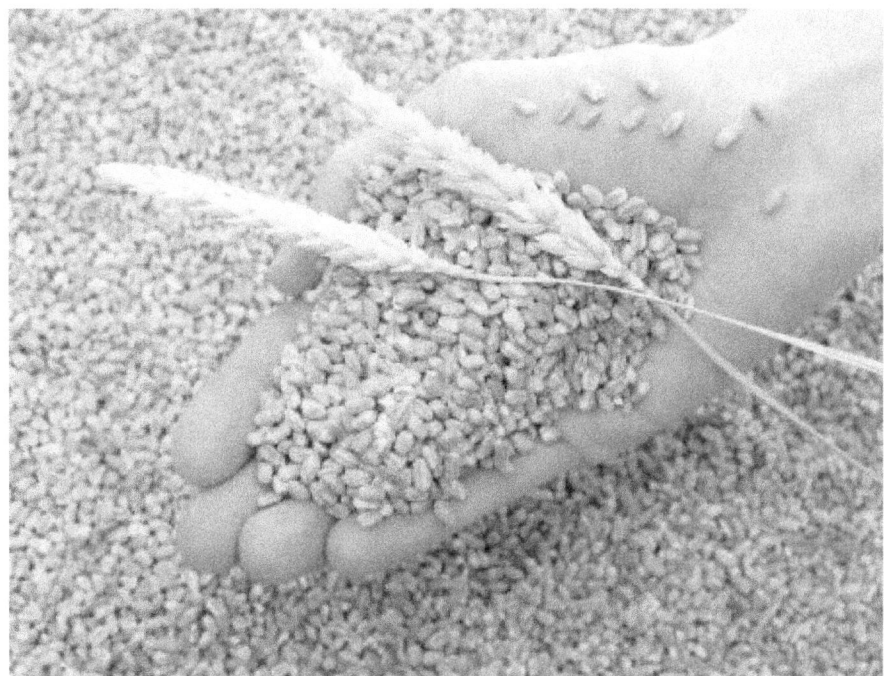

The color can be anywhere between golden brown to light tan in color depending on the variety and the type of the wheat strain.

Come to think of it, wheat is a cereal, so why is it to being called wheat "berry" in the 21st century? It is not a berry. It is a grain. This misguiding and faintly silly nomenclature by some foolish non-botanist for a grain of wheat is gaining popularity, but then he does not know that the term "berry" is used more often for fruit with an external skin covering, an inner stone and fleshy portion.

Wheat does not have a stony pit. Instead, it has a kernel. So next time somebody says "wheat berry" tell him the term is not correct. This is going to be as foolish as somebody starting to call a flower bud a "capsule" and fruit are going to be called nuts .[1]

So next time when you are talking about wheat, call a wheat grain a wheat kernel and not a wheat berry. Or, if you really want to differentiate between grain wheat and unrefined wheat, call the Golden grains wheat grains.

---

[1] Which means that if this ignorant misnaming and misleading trend continues you are going to be walking into the nearest florists' to ask for six pink rose capsules and then go to the nearest supermarket and ask them for a fresh supply of some cantaloupe nuts. I am surprised to see this terminology so prominent in Wikipedia , and also on about.com. Who thought this one up? Definitely not a scientist/researcher/botanist.

Nutritional Specifications of Wheat

Unaltered, unrefined wheat comes under one of the most naturally healthy items in the world. It is extremely rich in vitamins, minerals, and proteins, with 340 cal, in one serving and 73 g carbohydrates. This is 25% of what your body requires daily in terms of carbohydrates. It also has a high fiber content, which means that the more unaltered whole wheat you eat, the less chances you have of constipation.

It is very low in fat. That means you may eat as much wheat bread as you wish, and you are not going to grow chubby. B1, B2 and B3 are the vitamins which are present in the wheat in which bran and the germ has not been removed through refinement. The refining process removes 40% of the goodness from the wheat, and you have over refined glutinous flour, which is so commonly used for pastas and other baking products.

The difference between parboiled And Cracked Wheat

Bulgur or parboiled wheat is wheat, which has been semi-cooked. Cracked wheat is just crushed grains of wheat, which have not been treated in any manner of boiling and steaming to make them fit for human consumption.

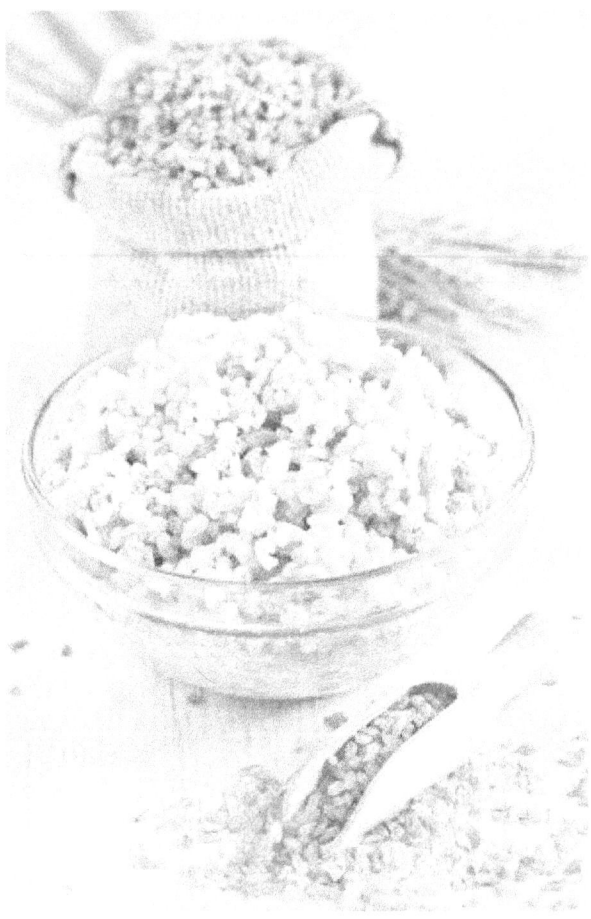

Raw and cooked bulgur

This bulgur is normally made without the removal of bran. That is why it is an excellent whole grain, which the USDA accepts as an edible and nutritious whole-grain.

This bulgur is easy to digest, that is why it is given to people who are recuperating from fever, ill, or have digestive problems due to age. The elders in the family in the East, Middle East, Armenia, Lebanon, Turkey, and even in many parts of the Mediterranean are fed bulgur based dishes to keep them healthy, fit and fine.

In fact my father, – who is in his 80s and just has a couple of teeth left – eats this parboiled wheat, – steamed once again in the pressure cooker with a little bit of water and preserved in the fridge in its soft porridge form – takes two handfuls of this bulgur, adds the cupful of creamy milk and a spoonful of sugar, gives it a boil and there he is, he has a healthy nutritious breakfast ready really quickly.

Easy to eat and to digest and he is getting his daily quota of the essential nutrients and vitamins required to keep the system functioning properly. And no, he does not suffer from constipation.

Bulgur pilaf is extremely popular in Middle Eastern cookery, so here is the recipe.

Our Daily Bread

Wheat is the staple grain diet in 60% of the world today. So, one wonders that if somebody had not crushed the grains of this wild grass, and extracted its flour to bake into bread more than 10,000 years ago, what would we be eating today?

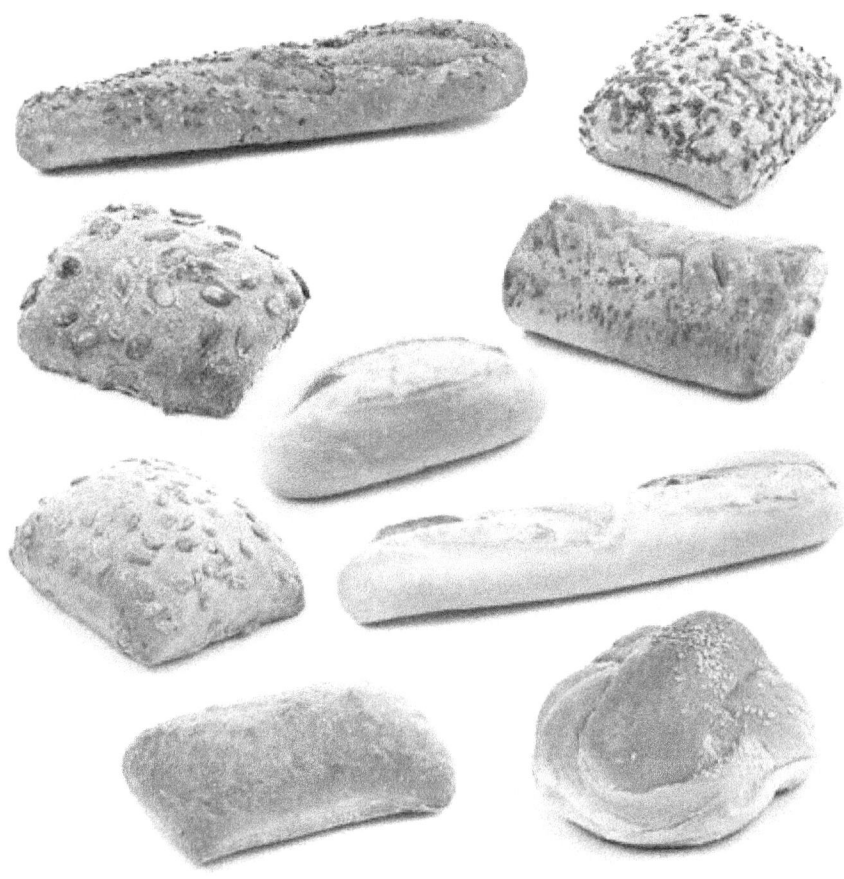

Living in an area, which was completely wheat oriented, throughout my life, it is not surprising that we took the role of wheat in Give Us Today Our Daily Bread for granted.

  One of the traditional things, which is slowly dwindling away in the hustle and bustle of the 21st century modern society is the hassled housemaker's skill in baking bread for the weekly consumption of her/his family.

Our grandmothers did not mind spending one whole day of a week in front of the hot oven, baking bread and other flour-based delicacies for the whole family. This was a tradition passed on from generation to generation. Or if she did not have the time to bake, she just used to slip over to the friendly neighborhood bakers and get freshly baked bread for grandpa's and her kith and kin's breakfast, lunch and dinner.

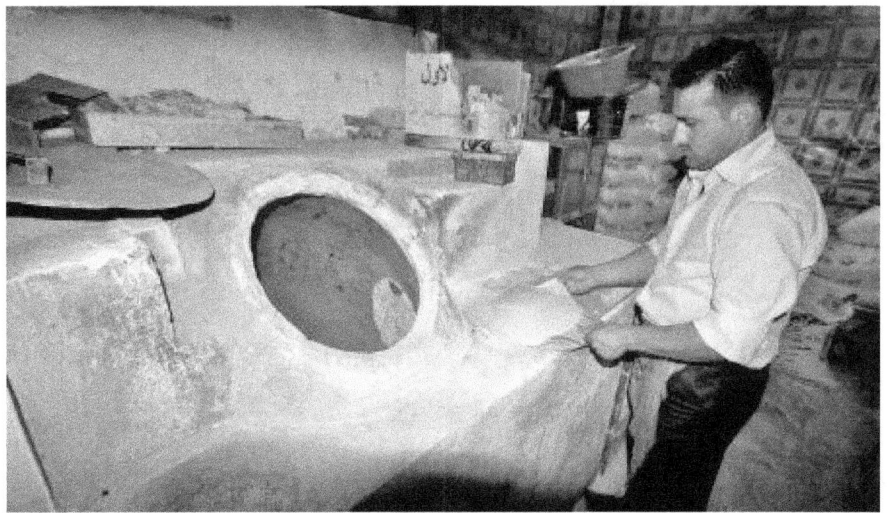

Thankfully, this taste for freshly baked bread has not been lost by us living in many parts of the world. Even today, if you find yourself walking down the lanes and streets of France, and many parts of Europe, you are going to see – let us say, the Parisians – coming out of the boulangerie (boo- lawn juhrry) with their fresh supply of spicy, herbal or garlic bread or baguettes to be enjoyed throughout the day.

Or they may be tempted with croissants, pastries, pies and cakes, freshly baked at dawn, and tempting you with their texture, flavor and fragrance. So would you. This tradition is not something new – it has been in vogue for millenniums in all the corners of the globe.

So is it surprising that homemade bread, which was once an important way of life, is coming into its own again, for all those people who think of good wholesome bread as an important part of healthy living.

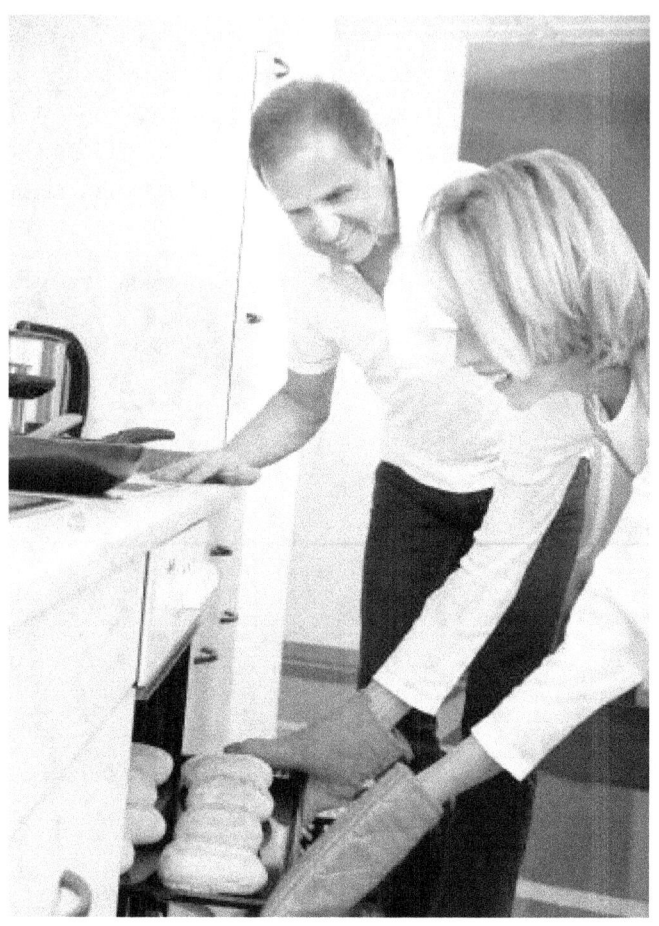

Nothing can beat the fragrance of freshly baked bread!

Plain White Bread

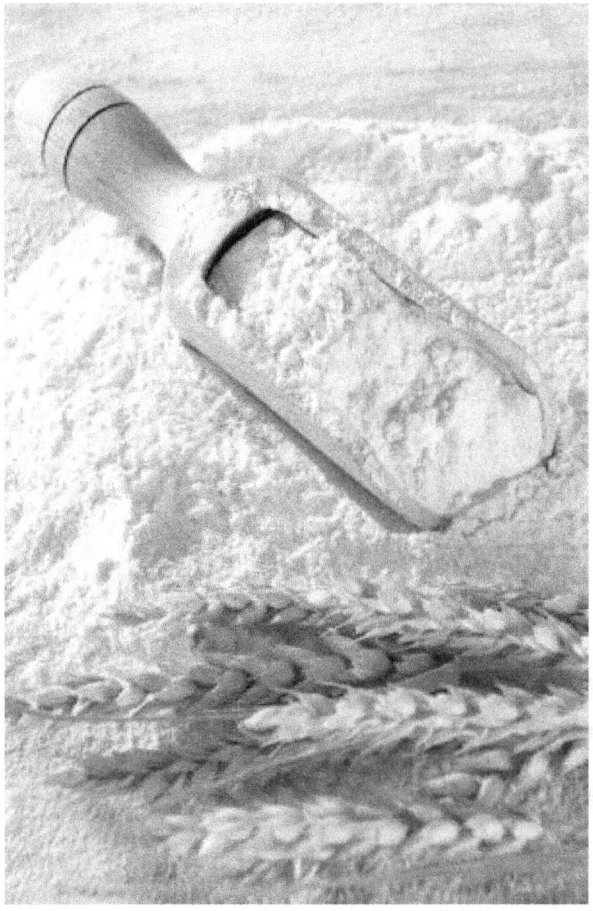

This bread is made traditionally, with flour, which has not been ultra-refined. So it is going to have bran in it, which is good for your digestion.

Nowadays, we may consider making bread to be lots of work, so I would suggest making about 3 pounds of bread at one time, and dividing it to be used as required.

You can freeze the baked bread or prepare the dough and then wrap it up in foil, and polythene to be baked when needed.

The ingredients needed to make that plain white bread, which caused revolutions to occur. And no Mary Antoinette did *not* say, "If they do not have bread to eat, let them eat cake." This was some malicious writer giving her bad press. But it was the lack of "pain" and the demand for it in plenty, which made her lose her head, figuratively speaking.

Bread and circuses was what the Roman public demanded more than 2000 years ago, baguettes and beurre,(*B uhrrrr*) – yes, that is butter in French – is what I want today. Made of highly nutritious, unrefined pure wheat flour.

So how do you begin making this bread?

Get the ingredients together –

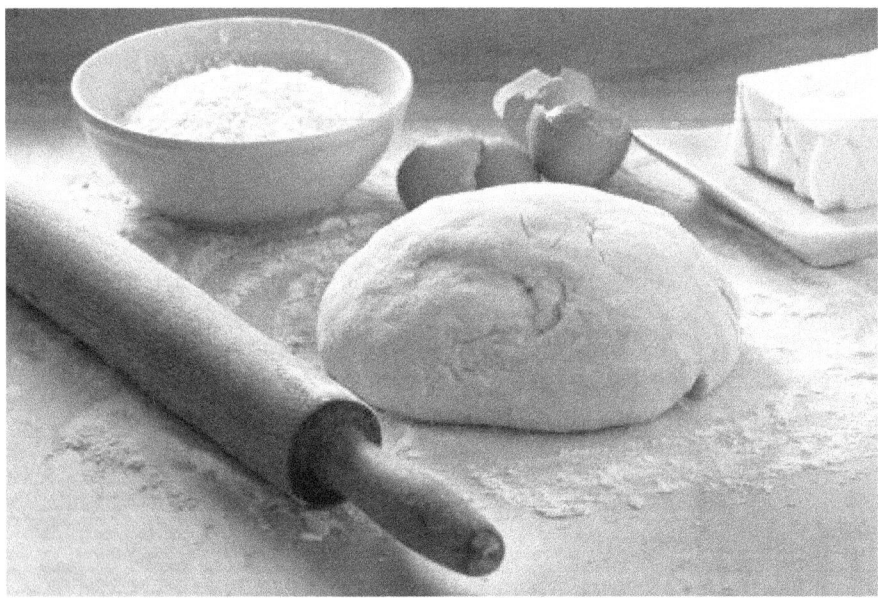

No, you do not need eggs, even though they are being used as a binding material. I am using butter for binding. Eggs can be used for glazing the crusty surface.

The traditional way of making it is to sieve 3 pounds of flour with no more than 1 ounce of salt into a large bowl. Rub in one – 2 ounces of butter or lard. Traditionally lard was used, but butter helps keep the bread crunchy and delicious tasting longer.

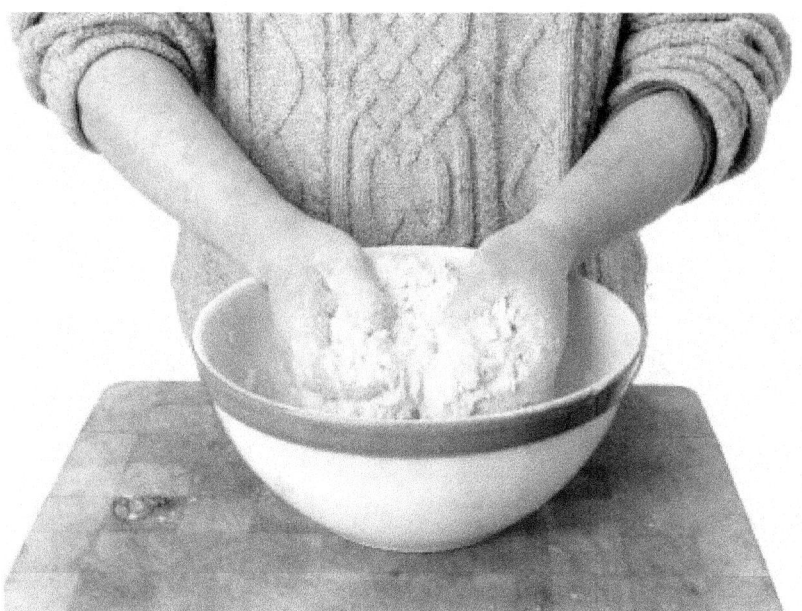

Warm one and a half pints of water to hand heat. That means it should be lukewarm, and your hand should not feel any discomfort when you dip it in the water.

Cream together 1 ounce of fresh yeast with a teaspoonful of sugar and warm liquid until it is runny, and leave for 2 to 3 minutes. This is if you are using fresh yeast.

If you are using dried yeast, mix with a little warm liquid, leave until it is frothy – 10 minutes.

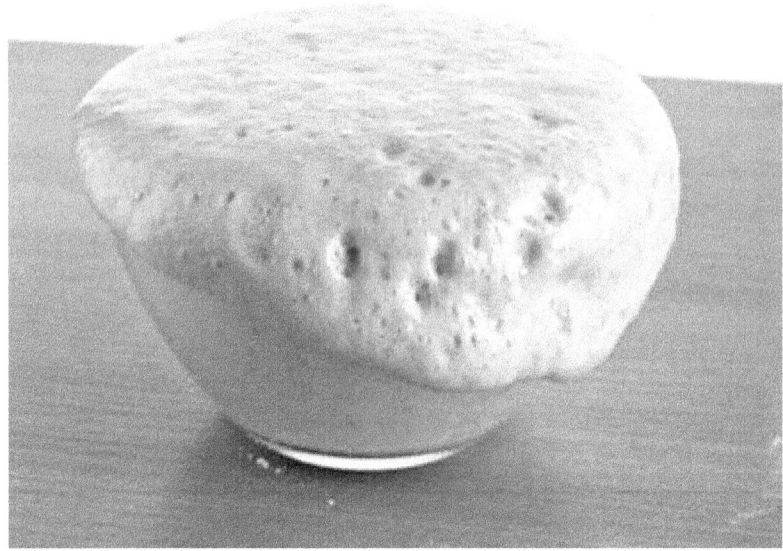

Add the yeast to the flour with the remaining liquid enough to give it a soft elastic consistency.

Start kneading the dough on a floured board by folding towards you, and pushing away with the heel of your hand.

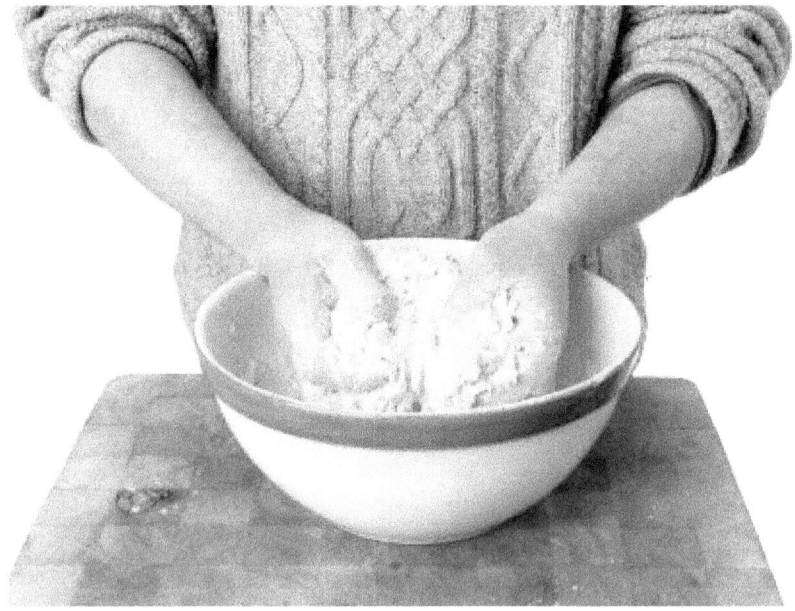

You need to knead this for 10 minutes to get the exactly right strength and help the bread to rise.

How Do You Get the Right Flour Consistency?

Press the dough lightly with a floured finger. If an impression remains, it should be kneaded even more.

In Asia and in many parts of the East, it is family tradition to start teaching children how to knead bread dough in order to make their daily bread, when they are very young. So by the age of seven, they know how to knead bread and bake it in the ovens, or on griddle pans.

In fact, the epitome of a well-trained Eastern traditionally well brought up domesticated girl is considered to be that girl who can knead bread in a kneading utensil[2], in such a manner that not a piece of wet or dried flour is left sticking to its sides.

---

[2] This high hipped, flat and big kitchen utensil is called a paraat and no kitchen can do without it in the East. This is how it looks and it is made up of either stainless steel or traditionally of bronze.

http://www.pankaj-boutique.com/en/indian-ustensils/2032-indian-container-paraat.html

I remember my favorite grand aunt admonishing me, after I had kneaded the dough, about 10 years ago. How come the paraat was in the sink, ready for washing? Had I made such a mess of the kneading process that I needed to *scrub* the sticky paraat? Had all these years of careful kitchen and culinary training still left me incapable of kneading dough properly? Horrors! Her sister-in-law, – my grandmother – had fallen down on the job of bringing me up properly, if I could not even clean up a paraat properly and left dough sticking to its sides. And so on and so forth...

Well, this is part of kitchen training in the East.

So, here is a tip for all those people who have instructors or relatives bugging you because of the sticky consistency of the dough while being kneaded. Push your fist to the kneaded dough before shaping it into a ball and leaving for proving. Take a spoonful of oil and spread it all over the surface of the paraat. Now use the fisted dough to figuratively wipe the floor and sides of the paraat. This removes all the sticky pieces of dough adhering to the sides. It also polishes the paraat, while giving the dough a good surface coating of oil. And it keeps the oldies / raised eyebrows happy!

This kneading dough tradition was also the one followed by grandmas in the West until women started breaking away with tradition in the late 20th century and began to consider learning how to cook to be old-fashioned stuff. And now many of them spend lots of money going to cookery classes to learn what they could have learned at their grandmothers' knee, just decades ago.

Naturally, this activity when done, for the first time is going to be fraught with danger, because we do not know about putting the right amount of water in the flour.

So when my grandmother dragged me protesting into the kitchen and told me that she intended to teach me how to knead bread, naturally, I did not bother much about looking at her sprinkling the flour with water and moistening it just enough, kneading that portion and then sprinkling more water in the rest of the flour and kneading it, in its turn.

I just tilted the water jug and the end result was a glutinous starchy mass thick and sticky enough to glue wallpaper. This can happen and this will happen for first time over enthusiastic cooks, kneading dough.

So, just keep plenty of dry flour handy. If the kneaded dough is too sticky, add some dried flour. The only problem is that you are going to end up with so much kneaded dough, that you have to preserve it in the fridge, depending on how much flour you got wet and sticky in the very beginning!

Put the dough in a greased mixing bowl, cover with an oiled polythene or a damp cloth. Allow it to rise by placing it in a warm place like an airing cupboard for one and a half hours, or at an average room temperature for about two hours or even in the refrigerator for 8 to 10 hours. The technical term is "prove."

This proven bread is going to rise because of the yeast. My uncle leaves it overnight, but then he learned that trick as a student in France, from his landlady.

She was one of the old school, who baked bread, fresh every morning and stuffed family, friends and tenants with oven baked goodies throughout the day.

Naturally, she being of the grandmother persuasion made sure that all her student tenants knew how to bake bread, because if they did not know that, there was something drastically wrong with their upbringing and their grandmothers!

Where have those days – and those good hearts – gone?

Uncle is the only one in the family who bakes homemade bread. The rest of us are too busy, alas, to do so. We promise ourselves that one day, we will do as he does, but as long as we have access to the nearest supermarket shelf and packaged day-old bread, we are going to grab it, on our way back home from the office.

So now your kneaded bread has risen to double its size and it is very soft. Knead it again.

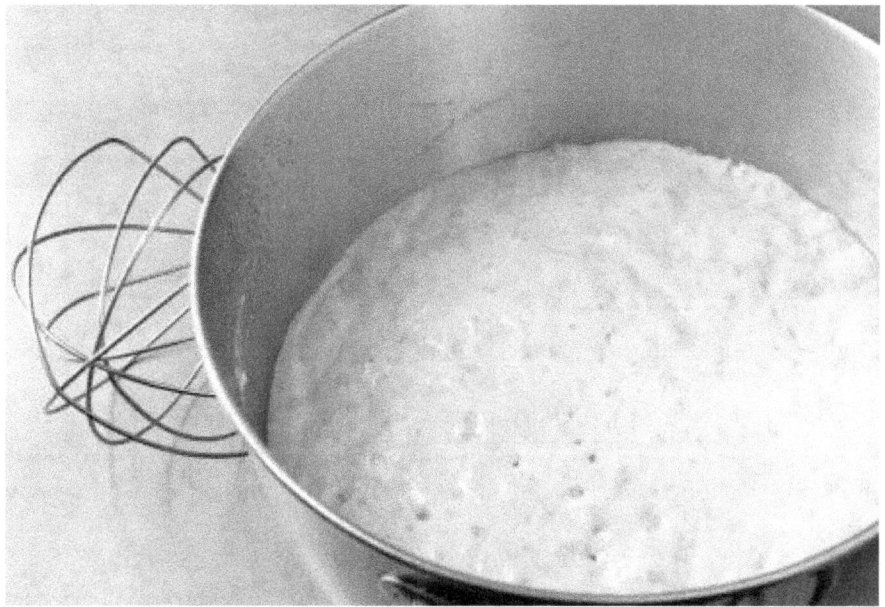

Turn on to a board, and needed, until it reaches to its original bulk. You do not need any dry flour now during this process. Test again with your finger to see it is sufficiently kneaded.

Shaping the Dough

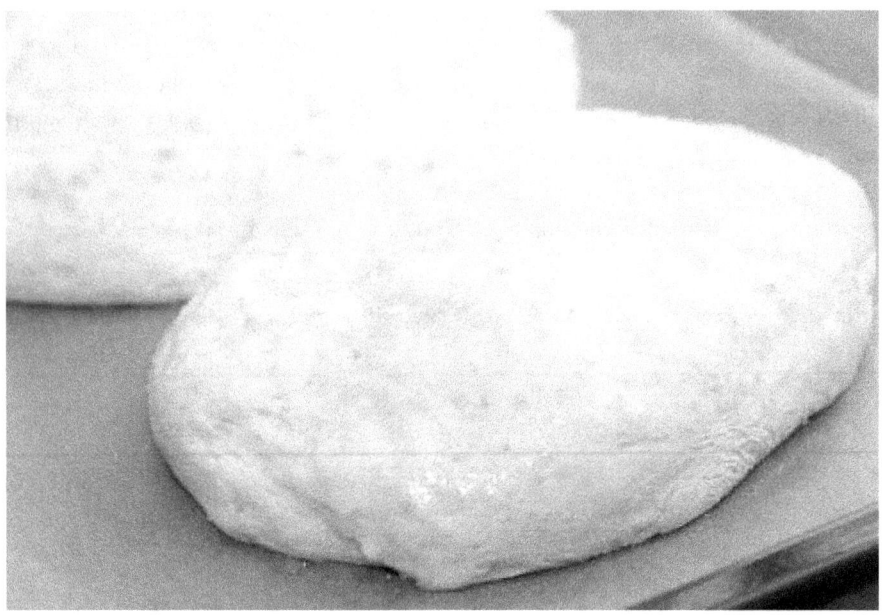

Divide the dough into three equal portions. Shape it into the shape you want.

To shape crunchy loaves, press 1 pound of dough into a large oblong, fold in three and put in greased, floured two pound tin. The crunchy upper crust is made by brushing the dough with an egg and sprinkling with cracked wheat or poppy seeds.

Put on a greased and floured baking tray. Cover loosely and leave to prove again until doubled in size. Then bake at 425°F for about 55 minutes.

It can take up to one hour and 20 minutes, depending on the temperature of the oven and the shape and the size of the bread.

Making Plaits

Roll the dough, into a long sausage. Flatten, cut in three strips, leaving one end attached. Plait. Prove, bake for 40 to 45 minutes.

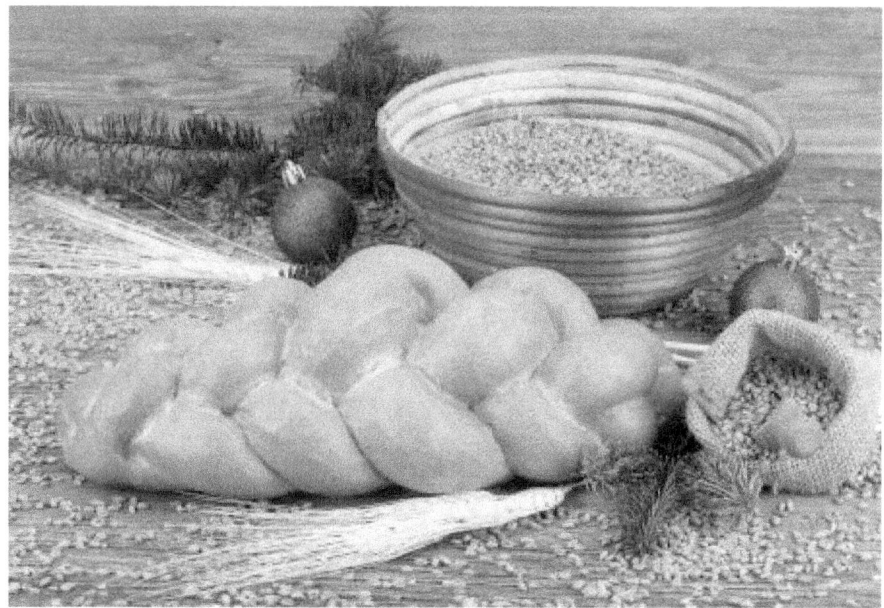

Dinner Rolls

Divide any remaining dough into two, divide one piece into eight and shape into traditional rounds, four – 5 inches fingers or tiny cottage loaves. Glaze top with egg and finish , and finish with a dusting of flour. Prove. Bake for 20 minutes.

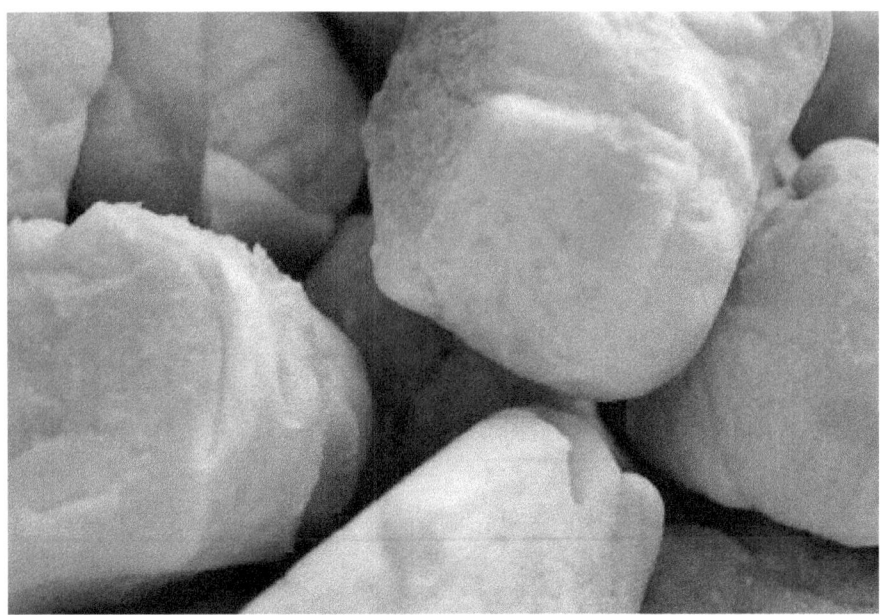

Mini cottage loaves

You can also make mini cottage loaves by making a ball from 2/3 ounces dough, and a smaller ball with 1/3 ounces. Place the smaller one on top and press the floured finger through to see both the balls.

Testing the bread

Knock the base of the loaf and the bread should sound hollow. Cool on wire rack, away from a draught. Do not preserve in the fridge – preserve in a bread box, after you have wrapped it up well.

Making a Cheese Loaf

I do not restrict myself to just grated cheese as a filling for this cheese loaf. Instead, I make up a mixture of garlic salt, scissored herbs, spices and grated cheese as a filler for this delicious cheese loaf.

Stretch out the dough with the help of a rolling pin in an oblong shape. Almost cover the oblong dough with your cheese spice mixture. Then roll, place in 1 pound tin which has been greased and floured, prove, and then bake for 30 to 35 minutes.

Perfect Bread Tips

You can use Baker's flour, which absorbs more heat we then will rise more. Plain flour has been used for centuries, but do not use refined flour. This refined flour has been processed in such a manner that it is going to become a solid glutinous mass sticking to the innards of your stomach and intestines because it has no fiber content.

Yeast must be really fresh. Traditionally, the yeast from last week or yesterday's baking is going to be used, but if you are starting for the first time, use baker's yeast bought from your nearest baker. If you are using dried yeast, it is going to keep well, if it is hermetically sealed, but it should not smell musty.

Fresh yeast should be a creamy – putty color and should crumble easily.

This yeast keeps in fridge up to three weeks, and in the freezer up to two months.

Have the ingredients and utensils warm, if your kitchen is cold to speed up the proving process. You can place the dough in a warm place near your stove to help with the yeast proving.

Be careful not to over prove or overripe dough. This gives the yeast a chance to give the bread yeast flavor and smell. The texture is also going to be coarse and chewy, unless of course you like yeasty bread.

More Traditional Wheat Dishes

Down the centuries, we have been using wheat, either in flour form to make our bread, or we have used the wheat kernels in broken form. This is called bulghar after it has been dried and crushed. Semolina is also a wheat preparation made up of coarsely ground wheat milled. Other wheat products which you are going to obtain after milling, apart from flour includes middlings and groats.

Groats are also known as bulgur or Dalia after raw wheat kernels have been steamed or parboiled. After that, they are crushed and the bran is removed from these dried wheat grains.

Just imagine that you went into an Egyptian kitchen 2000 years ago. You would be given bread loaves, made up of corn and wheat baked in a hot oven. Then you went exploring in other parts of Africa or in the Middle East. You would have wheat beer to drink. You would eat flatbread baked on a flat surface. You would also eat Couscous, which is still a staple dish in many parts of Africa.

Germinated wheat is used to make malt (that is the base for malt whiskey). At and crushed, you would get cracked wheat.

So this is the wheat, which you eat in the form of porridge, bread, doughnuts, pasta, rolls, pastries, muffins, biscuits, and also in shredded wheat and other breakfast cereals.

You need to have at least hundred grams of wheat every day to get a major part of your nutritional requirements. The world's favorite staple food is, of course wheat, along with rice. In fact, I have seen it growing 13,000 feet above sea level in Tibet, which shows you how mankind cannot do without this satisfying, healthy, nourishing blessing of nature.

The common varieties of wheat grown all over the world are red and white varieties, but there are places where you can get blue, yellow and black naturally evolved wheat species.

Raw wheat is definitely not edible, and it has to be sprouted, cooked, boiled, baked or prepared in any other way in order to be good for human consumption. Even though cooking lessens the nutritional content of cereals, it still has enough of protein and other important essential nutrients to keep you healthy, fit and fine.

Bulgur Pilaf

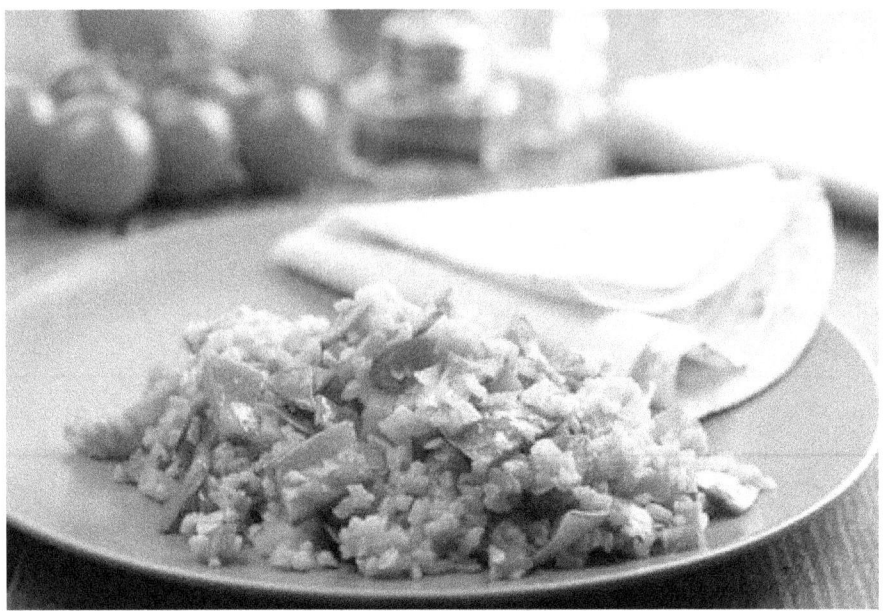

I am not using rice here. The moment you hear the word pilaf, you immediately get a vision of basmati rice steaming hot with pieces of meat and spices. This bulgur pilaf is cooked with onions, tomatoes and red pepper along with chicken stock.

Get these ingredients together –

1 cup large grained Bulgur, drained after washing.
2 cups freshly made hot chicken broth. [Learn how to make original traditional chicken broth in the <u>Appendix</u>].
If you do not have chicken soup ready at hand, just put one chicken bouillon soup cube in 2 cups of hot water.
One green pepper, one medium-sized onion, one medium-sized tomato, two leeks – scissor them well, instead of chopping and dicing them.
One teaspoonful of salt. That is only if you are using chicken soup. If you are using bouillon, it is already salted so use half a teaspoonful of salt.
One tablespoonful of butter
Sauté the onion until it is golden brown in the butter. Now add the green pepper, leek, tomato, salt, and the chicken broth. The chicken broth, which I made had

plenty of other vegetables in it, so I did not mind adding it to the pilaf, along the broth. The more the merrier.

When the water starts to bubble, add the bulgur and stir.

Half cover the utensil with a lid and cook on low heat until the water evaporates.

This is an exceedingly delicious and nutritious dish, which you can have for lunch. You can also eat it as a side dish with chicken dishes. I found it delicious with yogurt and water, -either served whipped till frothy with salt and pepper in a glass- or just yogurt with some chopped cucumbers, onions and tomatoes added. Use your own creativity to make this healthy meal.

Tabbouleh- Tabouli Salad

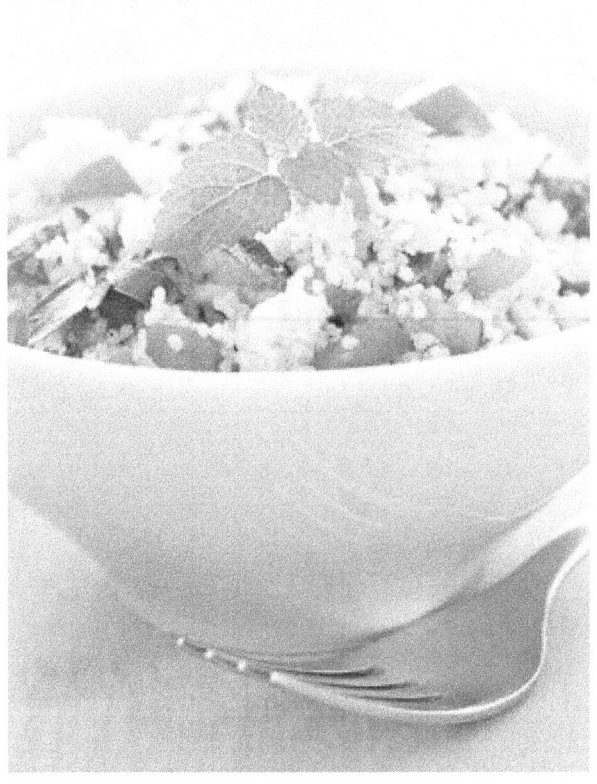

A Middle Eastern lunch without Tabouli salad would look incomplete.

You make this salad by collecting ¼ cup bulgur, 1 cup water, three green onions or leeks, one large tomato, one bunch of parsley scissored fine, juice of one lemon, half a cup of olive oil, mint for garnishing and salt and pepper to taste.

Immerse the bulgur in the hot water while you are preparing the other ingredients. This immersion is going to soften up the bulgur, while you are cutting and scissoring all the rest of the vegetables in a large bowl. Chop the tomato, onion, and the parsley. Add the olive oil, lemon juice, pepper and salt, and the mint.

Drain the water from the bulgur and put the wheat in the vegetables/oil mixture in your bowl. Mix with a large spoon. You can also add any other seasonal vegetables, herbs and spices, taken from your garden and enjoy with chopped cabbage leaves, lettuces, spinach leaves, forked up on your plate. Healthy, nourishing and tasty.

Finally ground bulgur is normally used to make another salad, just like tabouli, called Kisir. Here, you add fresh tomatoes, to my database, parsley, cucumbers, olive oil, and like I said, any other salad greens, which you want to add, depending on your personal taste.

Frumenty

Do not think that cracked wheat based dishes were just restricted to the East down the centuries. In the West, also, especially in Greece and Western Europe, this ingredient was a necessary part of medieval and ancient cuisine. Frumenty is one such dish, the name being derived from the Latin word for grain – *"frumentum."*

Depending on the area where you are eating Frumenty in Western Europe today, you are going to have different recipes, which may either be salty with broth, eggs and milk or sweet with sugar, almonds, orange flower extract, saffron, currants, and other dry fruit.

Frumenty was eaten all over Europe, especially during Lent, and as a traditional Christmas dish and also on special occasions, when it was considered to be a "subtlety" – a special delicacy.

Frumenty is considered to be one of the original dishes passed down from the Celtic times to modern times, and that is why it is called the oldest traditional and national dish by the British.

Frumenty was made traditionally by boiling whole grains in water until they were soft and cooked. After that, they were boiled in milk and sweetened with sugar. Flavor was added in the form of spices and cinnamon.

Another traditional method says – *[I am writing this verbatim in 21st century English from the original medieval recipe.]*

Take wheat and pound it in a mortar well until you have broken off the husks and hulls. Now put it in boiling water until the seeds burst from the hulls and allow it to cool. Now take freshly made broth, and the milk of almonds, along with the sweet milk of a cow and allow it to cook. *[Broth? Is this the dish salty, because as far as I know broth is made up of animal protein and vegetables?]*

Temper it with yolks of eggs, and boil a little. Allow to cool and then serve, ith fresh mutton and fat venison.(*All right, yes, this dish is salty. It is being used as a soup side dish with meat on Christmas.*)

Cous-cous

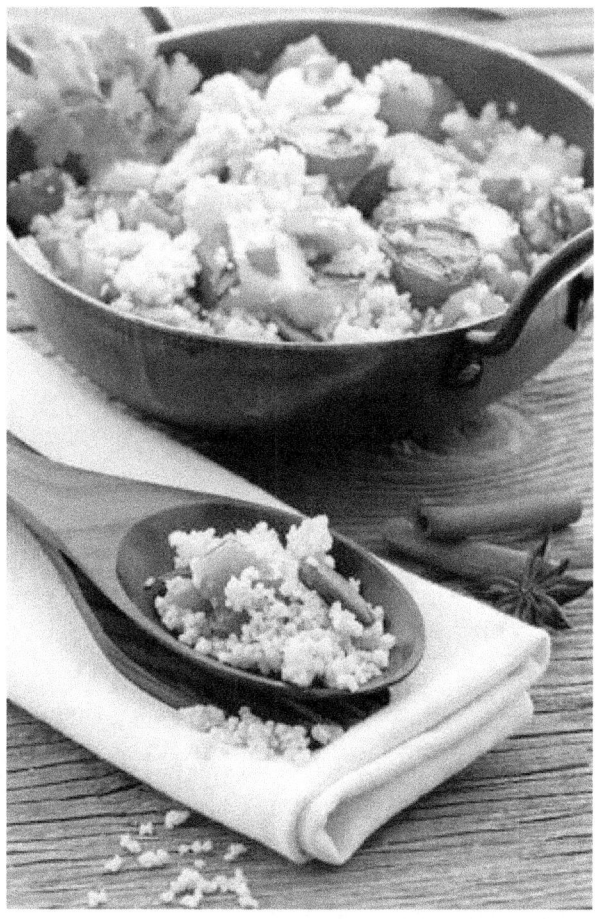

Cous cous is also a traditional dish, but instead of bulgur, it is made of semolina. It is extremely popular in North Africa, so I am indebted to this particular URL, which gave me a really good insight into the history of couscous. It is normally eaten with meat and vegetables.

http://www.cliffordawright.com/caw/food/entries/display.php/id/58/

All these nutritious wheat based items have been part and parcel of mankind's life, all over the globe. So anybody who intends to live healthy should add plenty of whole wheat based dishes to his diet chart right now.

Appendix

Traditional Chicken Soup

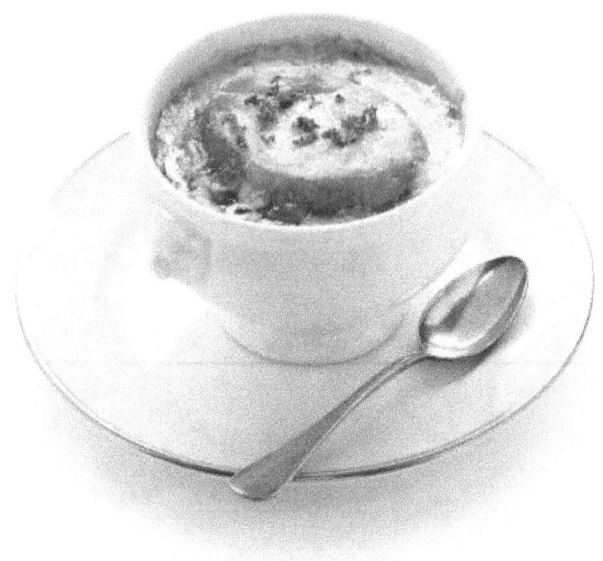

Traditional chicken soup, with fried pieces of bread? One of the most delicious and nourishing as well as comforting dishes which you can eat when you are tired.

2 pounds chicken, necks, backs and wings.

1 pound lean stewing beef, cut up in small pieces

1 pound soup bone – either veal or beef. [When I was buying this from the butchers, I told him that I wanted to make soup out of it, and he cracked it obligingly for me so that the marrow could add extra taste to the soup.]

¼ cup parsley, chopped coarsely

¼ cup tomato sauce. As this soup was taught to me by an Italian, no wonder it has tomato sauce in it. I just added some deseeded tomatoes also.

Two medium-sized carrots, left whole

Two stalks of celery, cut in 2 inch pieces

One green leek, cut into half inch slices up to the green part.

1 teaspoon salt, half full of pepper and 12 cups of cold water.

Put all of the ingredients in a large soup kettle and bring to a rolling boil. Use a slotted spoon to skim off the froth that is going to gather on the top. This froth is the vestige of fat, which was not removed from the lean meat.

Turn the heat back to simmer, cover and cook for three hours.

Strain the soup and pick out only the lean portions of the meat. Discard the rest of the meat because you have already extracted all the good from them.

Let this broth cool to room temperature, then put it in the coolest part of your refrigerator for several hours. Remove the hardened fat gathered on the top. Discard it.

You can either serve this soup as a clear broth before a meal, or use it to make bulgur pilaf. You may want to water it down with the addition of more water. This depends on your own taste and the type of meal you are going to serve it with. This quantity is enough for six people.

Panjiri- Pinnis

You may want to try this original traditional dish, which is definitely not for people with a sedentary lifestyle. Also, the large amounts of clarified butter was to get an unhealthy body back to its proper state of health.

This is a traditional dish for new moms in the northern part of the Indian subcontinent in order to keep them healthy[3].

---

[3] When I was born, my grandmother used to feed my mom a small bowl of Panjiri morning, evening and night, – not more than that – all the while she was nursing me. This is done to every mother in the North region of the Indian subcontinent. If her family could not afford Pinnis, the people of the village made them for her, down the ages.

Traditionally, the belief is the healthier the mother, the healthier the child. And so the tribe has healthy stock. So she was fed Panjiri three times a day regularly. If her health permitted, and she did not suffer from any reasons why she could not eat a high-protein diet food when expecting her baby, she would be fed this dish during the nine months of pregnancy and after, until she stopped nursing.

Statutory warning – if you are calorie conscious, do not touch this. The calorie count is in its high thousands.

Along with nursing moms, people who need plenty of heat and energy, especially in high-altitude areas breakfast regularly off this dish every morning. But then they are genetically inclined to assimilate all that protein. And their lifestyle is definitely not sedentary.

A long while ago, my brother demanded my grandmother make about 5 pounds of Panjiri to take back with him, for his breakfast and an energy snack, when he was posted at a high-altitude area. So she set him to grinding dry fruit, and edible gum and nuts and seeds and so helping her in the kitchen while she made about four packets of *panjiri* made into balls called *Pinnis.*

Each packet had about 10 baby fist sized pinnis and she calculated that that would serve him well for the next one and a half months.

When he rang up a week later, she asked him, "So how did your friends enjoy the *Pinnis*? I hope you shared some with them? "

The answer was a doleful, "I did not even manage to get one little taste of them. The moment I reached here, they started sniffing my baggage. Real honest to goodness homemade *Pinnis*, WOW, they yelled, and pounced. And finished everything, or just grabbed and ran before I could even say, hey, what are you doing, hands off. Next time let someone else's grandma make *pinnis* for those perpetually hungry wolves."

http://www.youtube.com/watch?v=0-g7YqX0HaY

This YouTube URL has English subtitles. You may want to look at the messages down below, where somebody has given the list of the ingredients.

It is a traditional dish, which is made up of wheat flour/semolina/wheat extract.

The dry fruit is, of course, very high in protein. Along with that the edible gum and the clarified butter makes this a very powerful dish, so you do not eat it if you are sick and your digestive system is not up to the mark. Or if you live in a hot area.

Conclusion

This book is a tribute to one of the most precious gifts of nature given to us – a golden grain of wheat.

Interspersed between information are some real-life anecdotes, about I, friends and foes, and all those people who have touched my life and added to my knowledge base.

All of the hilarious [and some not so hilarious] instances recounted in all my books are real-life episodes, narratives and incidents with real-life people like you and I. And if they – or I for that matter – act crazy impractical, or possibly plain weird at times, is not that what life is all about?

So live life Emperor size, live it healthy, Live Long and Prosper!

Check out some of the other Healthy Gardening Series books at Amazon.com

Gardening Series on Amazon

Author Bio-

Dueep Jyot Singh is a Management and IT Professional who managed to gather Postgraduate qualifications in Management and English and Degrees in Science, French and Education while pursuing different enjoyable career options like being an hospital administrator, IT,SEO and HRD Database Manager/ trainer, movie , radio and TV scriptwriter, theatre artiste and public speaker, lecturer in French, Marketing and Advertising, ex-Editor of Hearts On Fire (now known as Solstice) Books Missouri USA, advice columnist and cartoonist, publisher and Aviation School trainer, ex- moderator on Medico.in, banker, student councilor ,travelogue writer … among other things!

One fine morning, she decided that she had enough of killing herself by Degrees and went back to her first love -- writing. It's more enjoyable! She already has 48 published academic and 14 fiction- in- different- genre books under her belt.

When she is not designing websites or making Graphic design illustrations for clients , she is browsing through old bookshops hunting for treasures, of which she has an enviable collection – including R.L. Stevenson, O.Henry, Dornford Yates, Maurice Walsh, De Maupassant, Victor Hugo, Sapper, C.N. Williamson, "Bartimeus" and the crown of her collection- Dickens "The Old Curiosity Shop," and so on… Just call her "Renaissance Woman") - collecting herbal remedies, acting like Universal Helping Hand/Agony Aunt, or escaping to her dear mountains for a bit of exploring, collecting herbs and plants and trekking.

Our books are available at

1. Amazon.com
2. Barnes and Noble
3. Itunes
4. Kobo
5. Smashwords
6. Google Play Books

Check out some of the other JD-Biz Publishing books

Gardening Series on Amazon

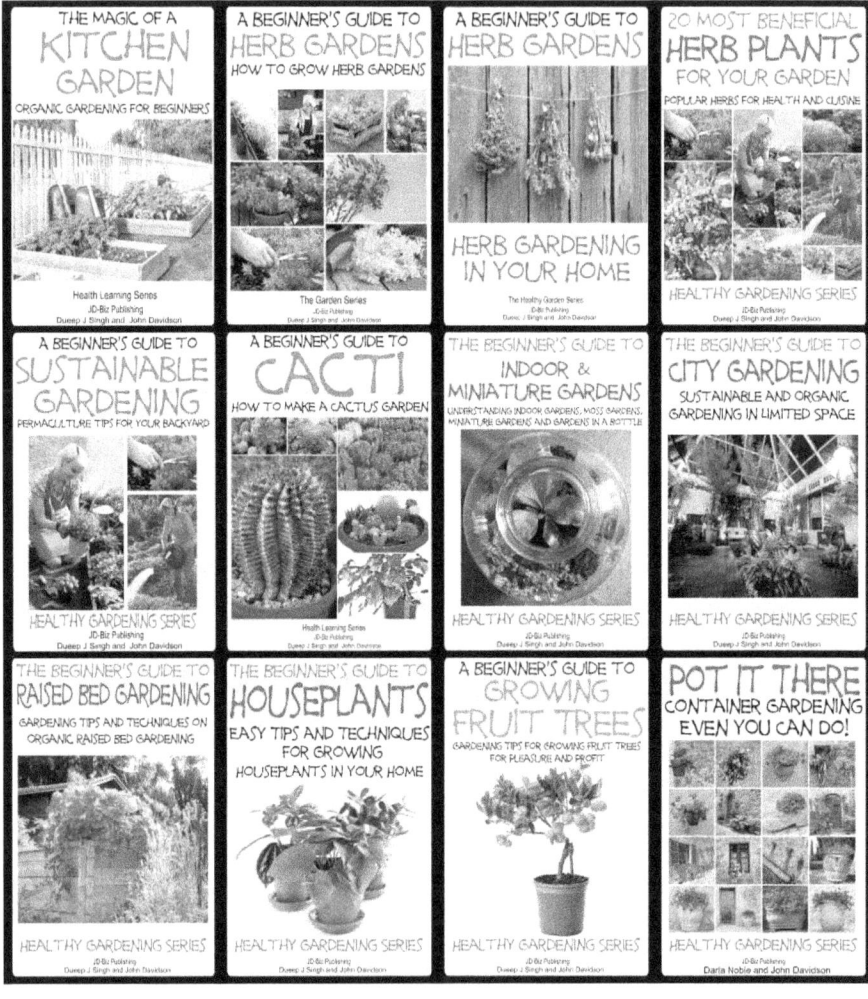

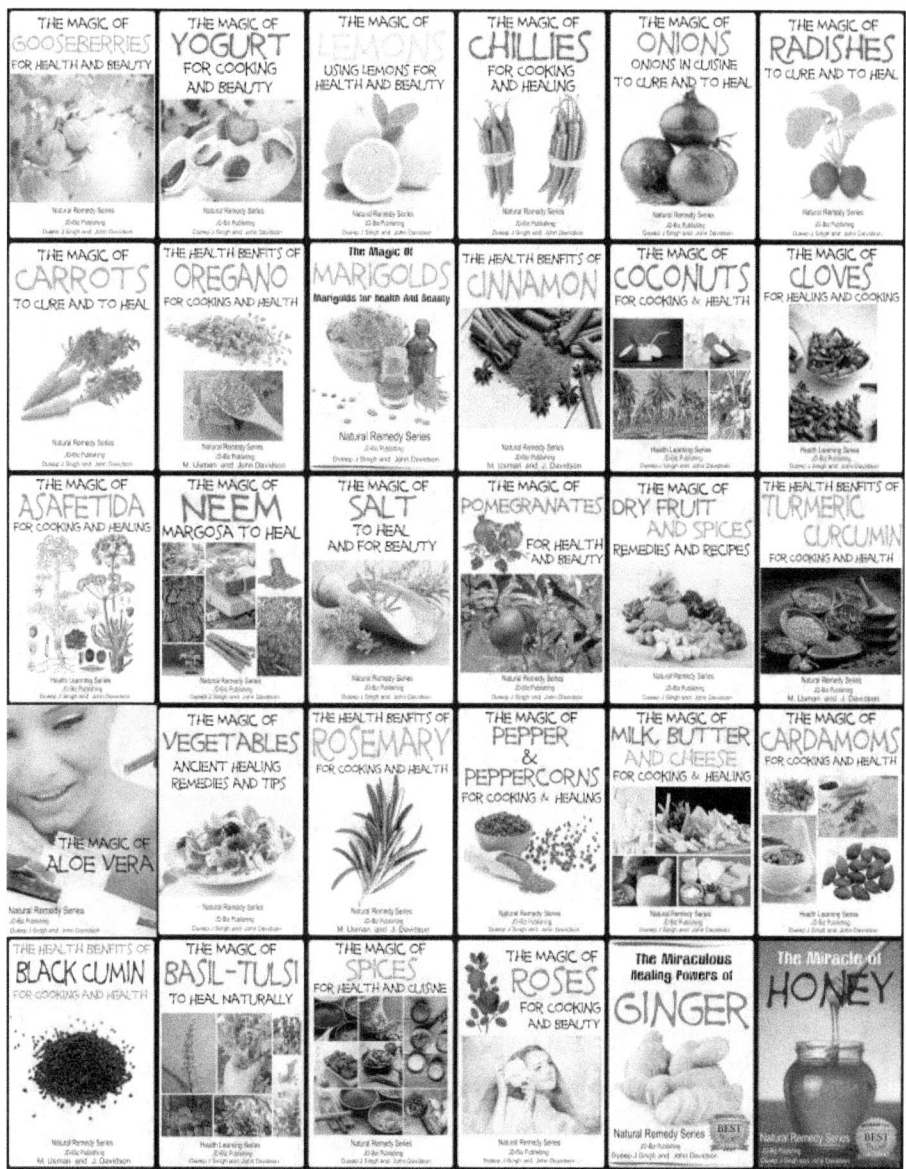

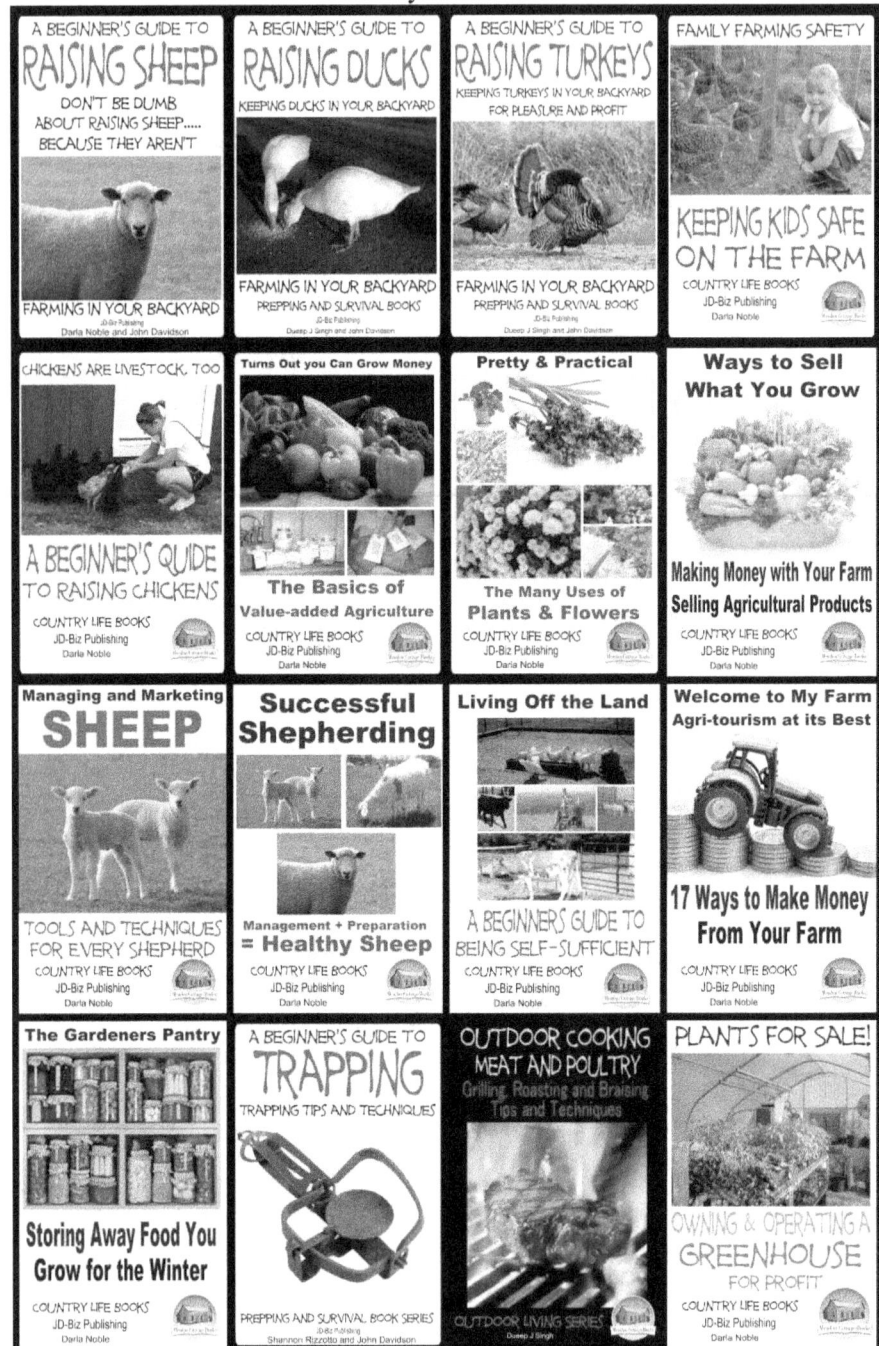

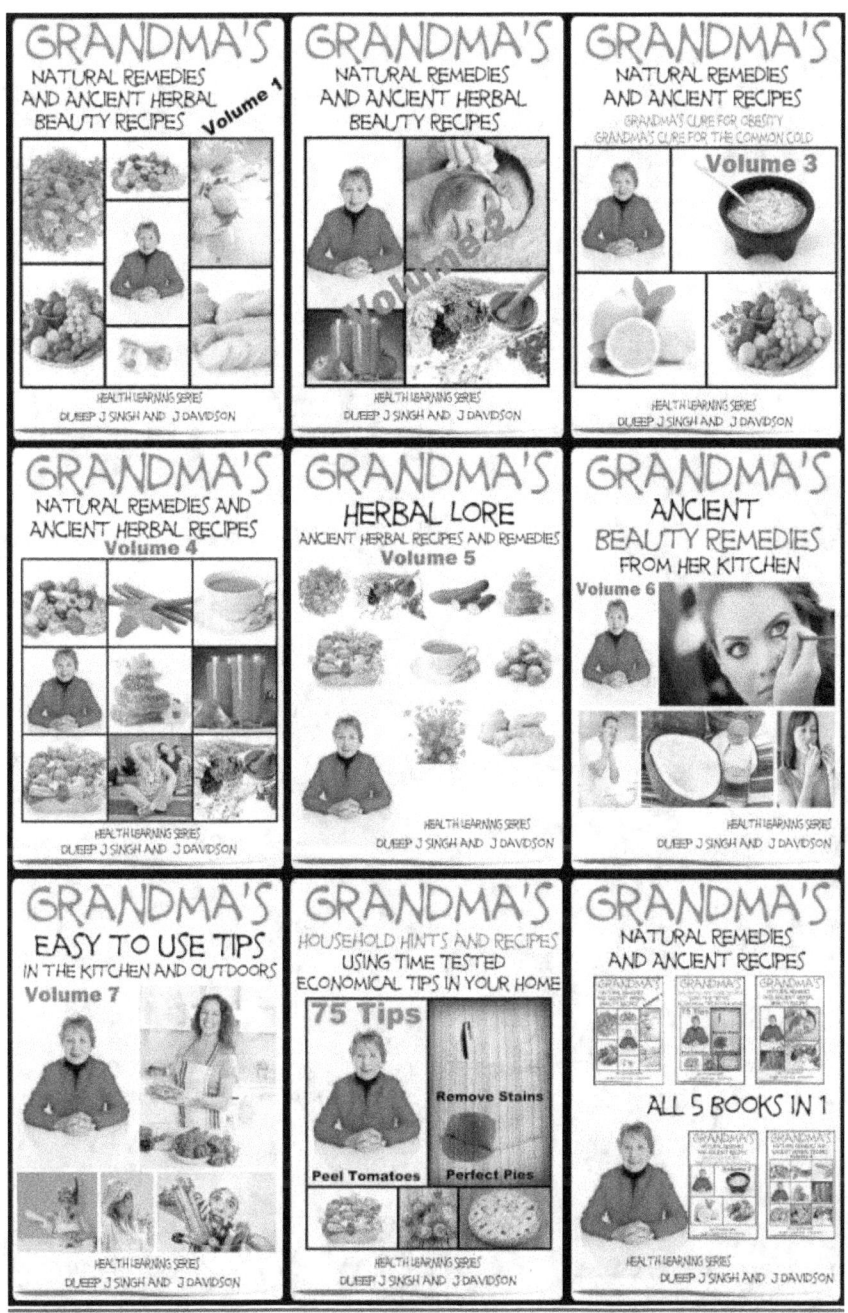

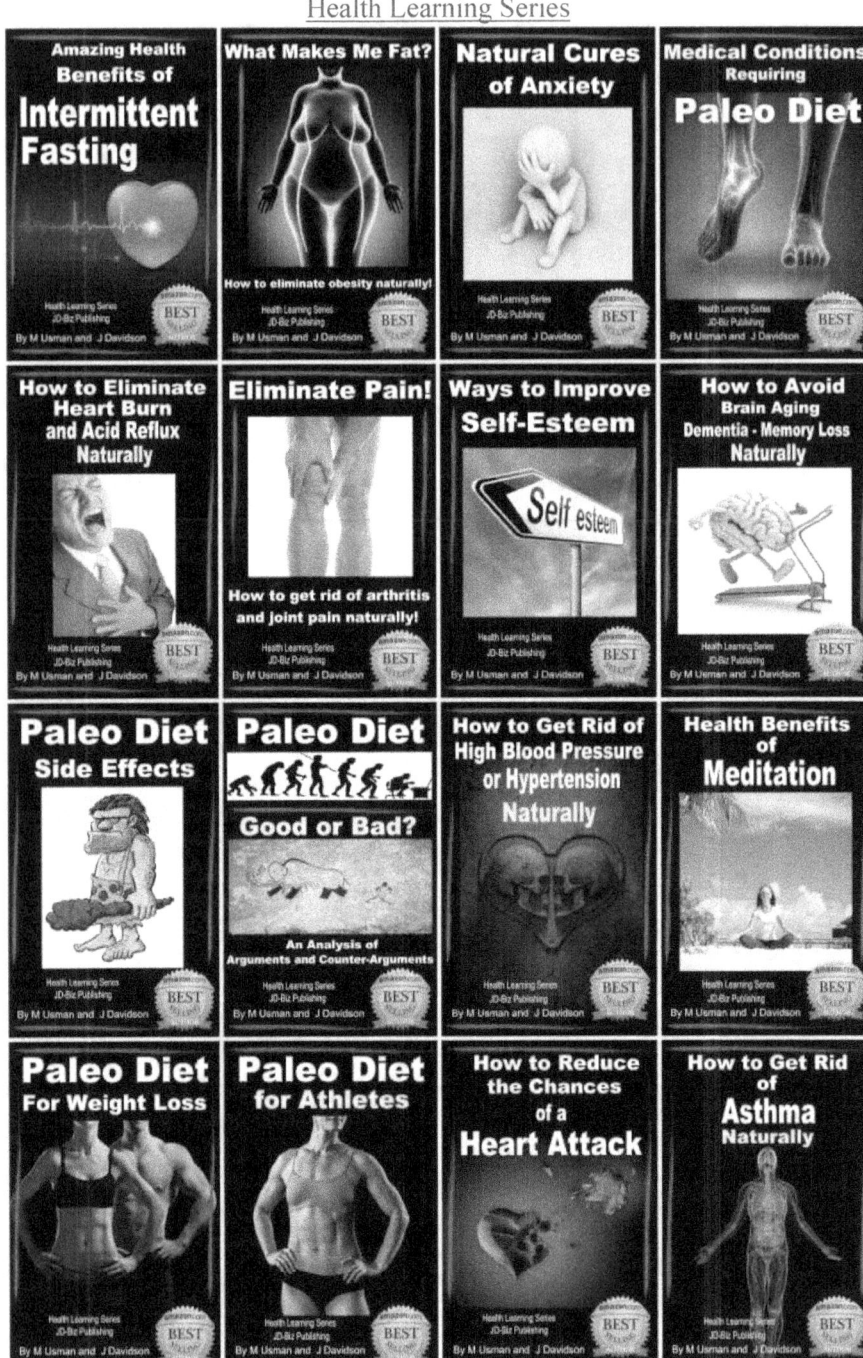

Amazing Animal Book Series

Learn To Draw Series

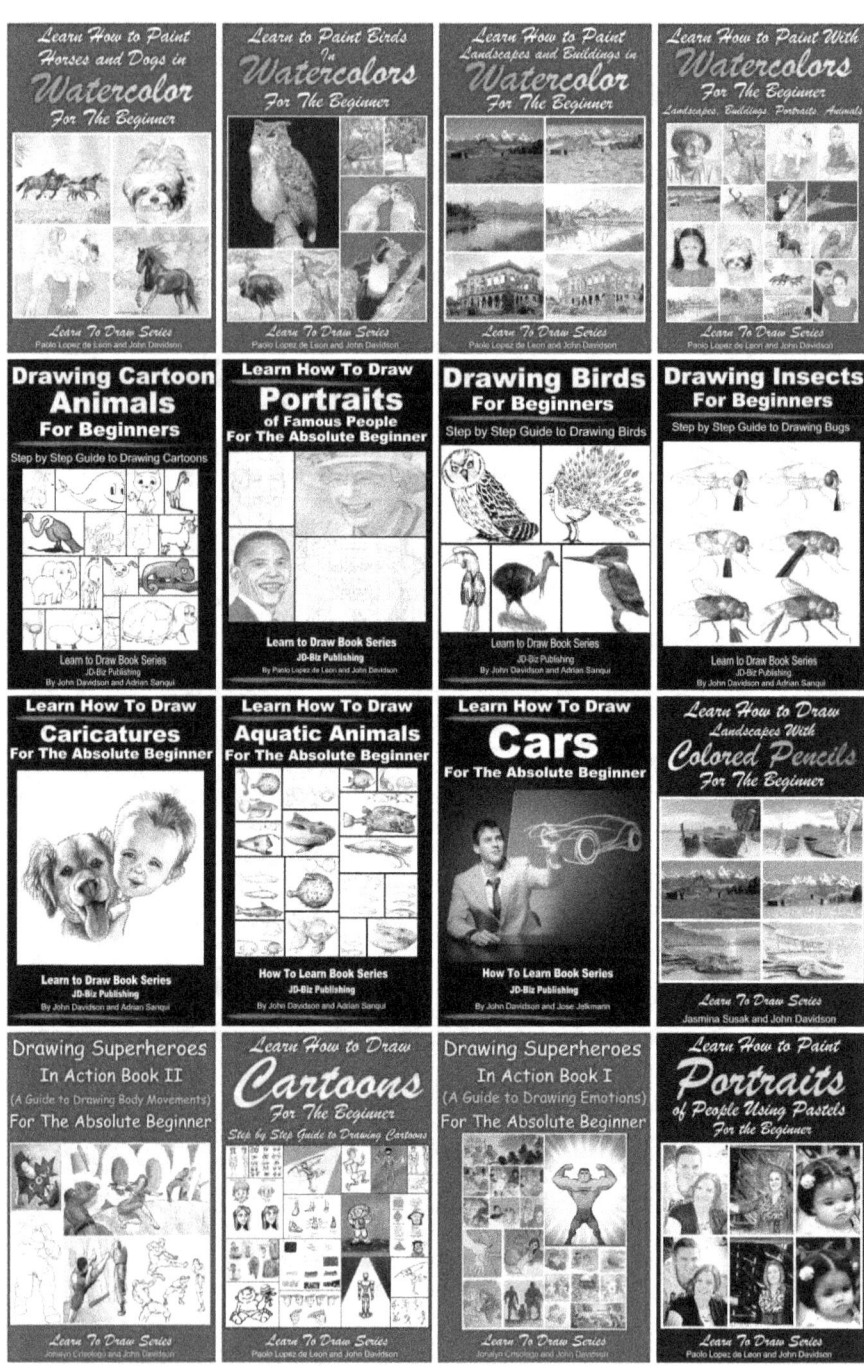

How to Build and Plan Books

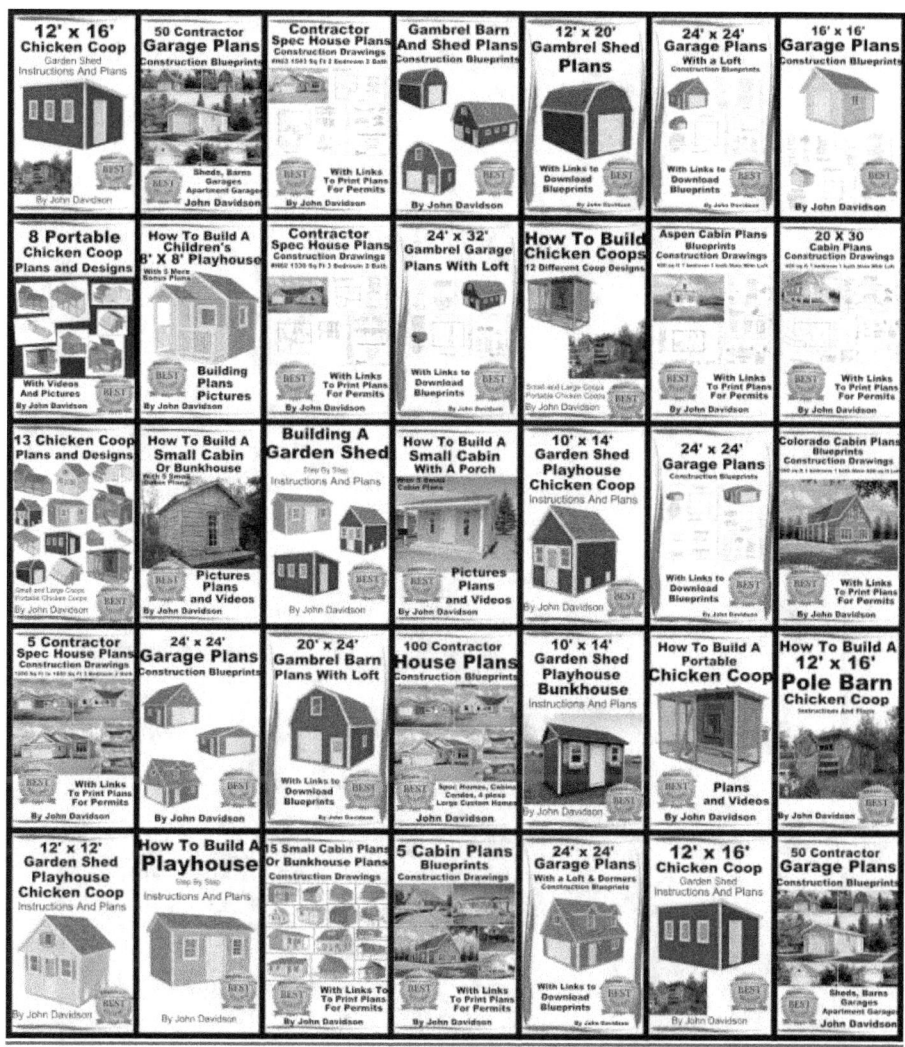

Entrepreneur Book Series

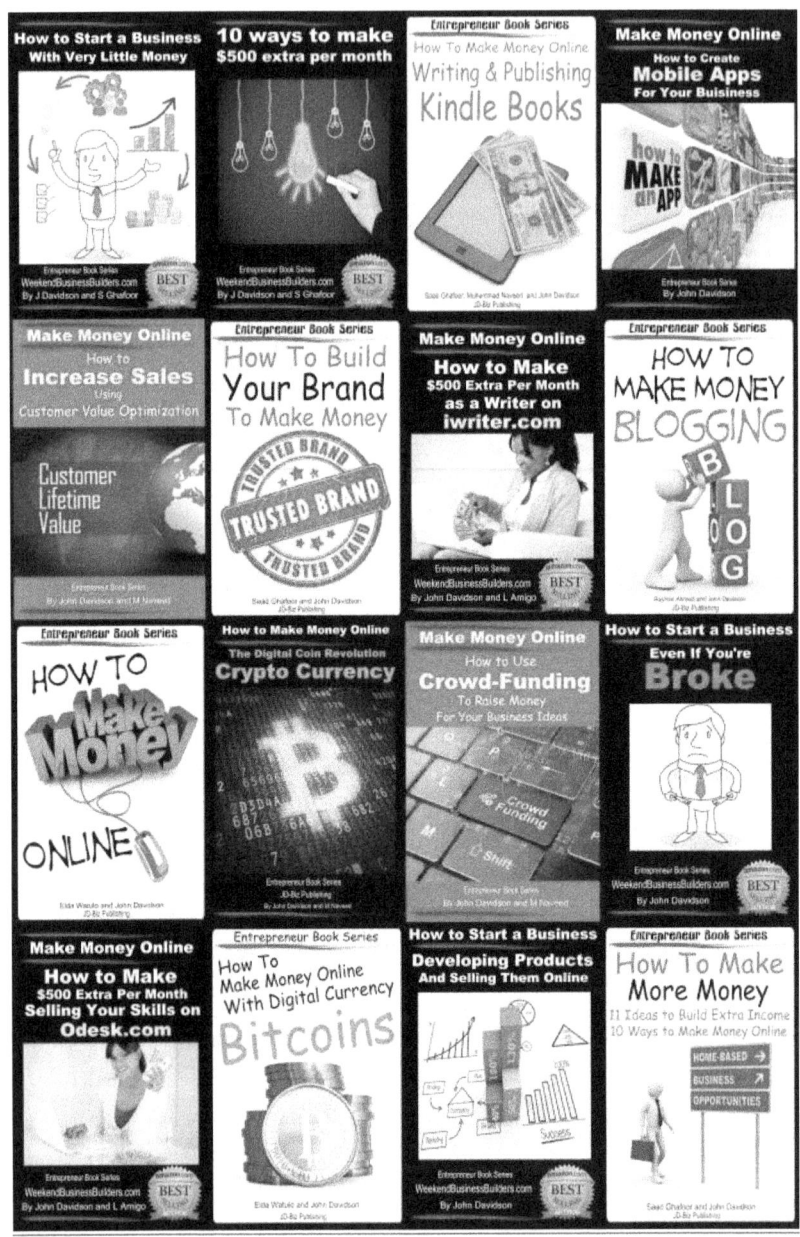

Publisher

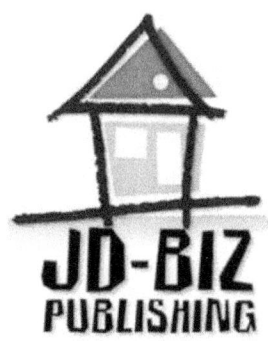

JD-Biz Corp

P O Box 374

Mendon, Utah 84325

http://www.jd-biz.com/

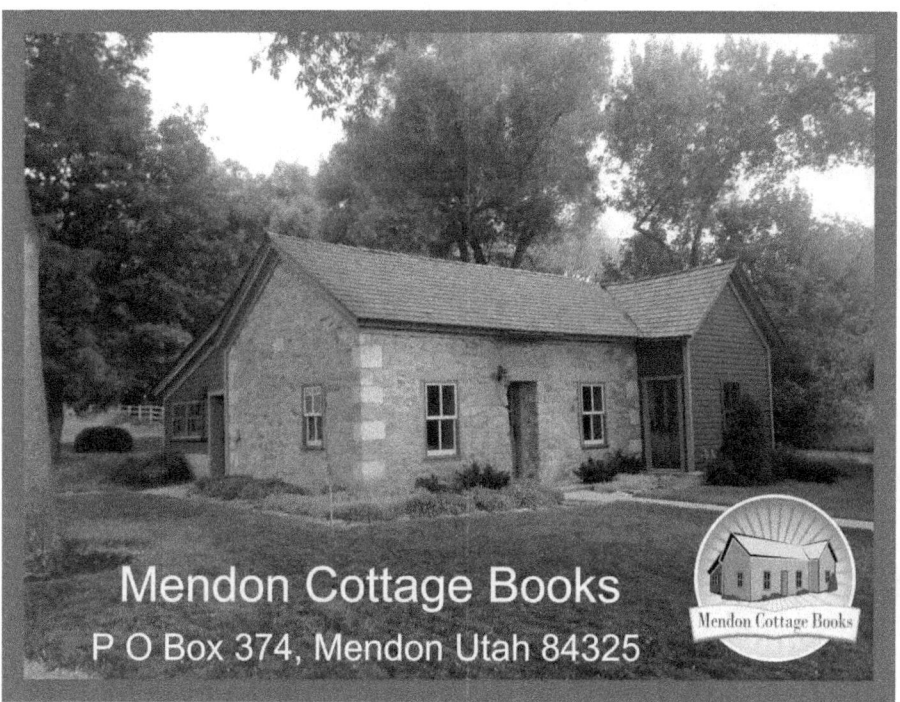